Tooth Health Beginners Guide

Lifestyle Factors Affecting Tooth Health

By

Brighton Conor
Copyright@2023

Table of Contents

CHAPTER 1

Introduction to Tooth Health

Oral health is a fundamental aspect of our overall well-being that often goes beyond the confines of a mere smile. It encompasses the health and hygiene of our teeth, gums, and the entire oral cavity. While the aesthetic value of a bright, healthy smile cannot be denied, the significance of maintaining good tooth health extends far deeper. We will delve into the importance of oral health and how it intricately interconnects with our overall physical and mental well-being.

1.1 Understanding the Importance of Oral Health

Oral health is not solely about preventing bad breath or cavities; it is a vital aspect of maintaining the proper functioning of our entire body. Our mouth is the gateway to our body, and the state of our oral health can have significant implications for our overall health. Numerous studies have shown a strong link between oral health and various systemic diseases, such as diabetes, cardiovascular diseases, respiratory infections, and even adverse pregnancy outcomes.

One of the key reasons oral health matters is that the mouth is teeming with bacteria. While most of these bacteria are harmless, some can contribute to the development of dental issues like cavities and gum disease. Proper oral hygiene practices, including regular brushing, flossing, and visits to the dentist, help control the growth of harmful bacteria and prevent these issues from escalating.

Beyond the physical aspect, oral health also has psychological and social dimensions. A healthy smile can boost self-confidence and improve social interactions. On the contrary, oral health problems can lead to embarrassment, reduced self-esteem, and even social isolation. This highlights the impact oral health can have on our mental and emotional well-being.

1.2 How Good Tooth Health Affects Overall Well-being

The connection between oral health and overall well-being is a dynamic and symbiotic relationship. Here's how good tooth health positively influences different aspects of our well-being:

Digestive Health: The digestive process begins in the mouth, where enzymes in saliva initiate the breakdown of food. Healthy teeth enable efficient chewing, which aids in proper digestion and nutrient absorption.

Nutrition: A healthy mouth allows us to enjoy a diverse range of foods, including fruits, vegetables, and proteins. Painful teeth or gum issues can limit food choices, potentially affecting our nutritional intake.

Speech and Communication: Teeth play a crucial role in forming sounds and speech. Well-maintained teeth enable clear and effective communication, contributing to social and professional interactions.

Pain Prevention: Dental problems can cause significant pain, affecting our ability to focus on daily tasks. Toothaches or discomfort can lead to disrupted sleep and reduced quality of life.

Cardiovascular Health: Emerging research suggests a link between gum disease and cardiovascular diseases. Bacteria from gum infections might enter the bloodstream, potentially contributing to inflammation in the arteries.

Diabetes Management: Gum disease can make it harder to control blood sugar levels in individuals with diabetes. Conversely, uncontrolled diabetes can impair the body's ability to fight oral infections.

Pregnancy Outcomes: Pregnant individuals with poor oral health are at an increased risk of preterm birth and low birth weight. Hormonal changes during pregnancy can also exacerbate oral health issues.

In essence, our mouth serves as a mirror reflecting our overall health status. Neglecting oral health can have far-reaching consequences that extend beyond toothaches and cavities. Conversely, prioritizing oral hygiene and seeking regular dental care can contribute to a healthier, more vibrant life.

Understanding the significance of oral health lays the foundation for the subsequent sections of this guide, which will delve into the intricacies of maintaining good tooth health, preventing dental issues, and embracing habits that support both oral and overall well-being.

CHAPTER 2

The Anatomy of Teeth

Teeth are remarkable structures that play a crucial role in our daily lives, enabling us to bite, chew, speak, and smile. To fully appreciate the importance of tooth health, it's essential to understand the intricate anatomy of teeth. We will explore the different types of teeth and their functions, as well as the complex structure that lies beneath the surface.

2.1 Different Types of Teeth and Their Functions

Human mouths house a variety of teeth, each uniquely designed to perform specific functions in the process of mastication and overall oral function. The three main types of teeth are incisors, canines, and molars.

Incisors: These are the front teeth and are characterized by their sharp, chisel-like edges. Incisors are used for cutting food into smaller, manageable pieces. They play a significant role in the initial stages of digestion.

Canines: Canines are slightly pointed and are often referred to as "eye teeth." They are well-suited for tearing and gripping food. Canines are crucial for biting into and holding onto foods before the molars take over the task of grinding.

Molars: Molars are large, flat teeth located at the back of the mouth. They have broad surfaces with ridges that aid in grinding and crushing food. Molars are essential for breaking down food into smaller particles that are easier to digest.

Premolars (Bicuspids): Positioned between the canines and molars, premolars have a flatter surface than molars but still contribute to grinding and tearing food. They have two or more pointed cusps, which is why they are sometimes referred to as bicuspids.

Each type of tooth works in harmony to facilitate the entire chewing process, ensuring food is broken down into digestible components. A balanced dental arch consists of a combination of these tooth types, each contributing uniquely to oral function.

2.2 Tooth Structure: Enamel, Dentin, Pulp, and Cementum

Beneath the visible surface of a tooth lies a complex structure that provides its strength, resilience, and functionality. Understanding the different layers of a tooth can help us appreciate the importance of protecting and maintaining its health.

Enamel: Enamel is the outermost layer of a tooth and is the hardest substance in the human body. It serves as a protective shield for the underlying layers. Enamel is primarily composed of minerals and is responsible for withstanding the forces of biting and chewing.

Dentin: Located beneath the enamel, dentin is a hard tissue that forms the bulk of a tooth's structure. It's not as hard as enamel but still provides strength and support. Dentin contains tiny tubules that transmit sensations like temperature changes to the tooth's nerve.

Pulp: The pulp is the innermost part of the tooth and contains blood vessels, nerves, and connective tissues. It plays a crucial role during tooth development but remains important throughout the tooth's life by providing nourishment and sensory functions.

Cementum: Cementum covers the tooth's roots and helps anchor the tooth in the jawbone through a network of fibers known as the periodontal ligament. It's not as hard as enamel but is essential for maintaining tooth stability within the jaw.

This intricate combination of enamel, dentin, pulp, and cementum creates a functional and resilient structure that allows teeth to endure the demands of daily use. It's important to note that while enamel is incredibly strong, it can still erode due to acids produced by bacteria and acidic foods. This erosion can lead to cavities and other dental issues, underscoring the importance of proper oral hygiene and regular dental care.

As we explore the various aspects of tooth health, remember that the anatomy of teeth provides the foundation for understanding how to

maintain their health and preserve
their function throughout our lives.

CHAPTER 3

Common Dental Issues

Maintaining good tooth health involves understanding and addressing common dental issues that can arise over time. We will explore some of these issues, their causes, prevention methods, and potential treatments, providing you with the knowledge to take proactive steps toward a healthier smile.

3.1 Tooth Decay (Cavities): Causes, Prevention, and Treatment

Tooth decay, commonly known as cavities or dental caries, is one of the most prevalent dental issues. It occurs when acids produced by bacteria in the mouth erode the enamel, leading to the formation of small holes or cavities. If left untreated, cavities can progress and cause pain, infections, and even tooth loss.

Causes: The primary cause of cavities is poor oral hygiene. Bacteria feed on sugars and produce acids that wear down enamel. Other factors include consuming sugary or acidic foods, frequent snacking, inadequate fluoride exposure, and dry mouth.

Prevention: Regular brushing and flossing are essential to remove plaque and food particles that contribute to decay. Limiting sugary foods and drinks, using fluoride toothpaste, and drinking fluoridated water can also help prevent cavities. Dental sealants, which are protective coatings, can be applied to molars to create a barrier against decay.

Treatment: Small cavities can be treated with fillings made from various materials, such as composite resin, amalgam, or porcelain. Advanced decay may require more extensive treatments like dental crowns or root canal therapy.

3.2 Gum Disease: Gingivitis and Periodontitis

Gum disease, also known as periodontal disease, affects the tissues surrounding the teeth. It ranges from mild gingivitis to severe periodontitis and can lead to gum recession, tooth loss, and even systemic health issues.

Gingivitis: Gingivitis is the earliest stage of gum disease and is characterized by red, swollen, and bleeding gums. It's usually caused by poor oral hygiene that allows plaque to build up along the gumline.

Periodontitis: Untreated gingivitis can progress to periodontitis, where the gums pull away from the teeth, forming pockets that can become infected. This infection can lead to bone and tissue loss, potentially causing teeth to become loose or fall out.

Prevention: Regular brushing and flossing, along with professional dental cleanings, are crucial for preventing gum disease. Managing risk factors like smoking, diabetes, and stress can also help reduce the risk of developing gum issues.

Treatment: Treatment varies based on the severity of the disease. Scaling and root planning are common procedures to remove plaque and tartar from below the gumline. In advanced cases, surgical interventions might be necessary.

3.3 Tooth Sensitivity: Causes and Remedies

Tooth sensitivity is a common issue that causes discomfort when teeth are exposed to hot, cold, sweet, or acidic stimuli. It occurs when the protective enamel is worn down, exposing the dentin and nerve endings.

Causes: Tooth sensitivity can result from enamel erosion due to tooth grinding, aggressive brushing, acidic foods, gum recession, or cavities.

Remedies: Using a soft-bristle toothbrush, practicing gentle brushing techniques, and using toothpaste specifically designed for sensitive teeth can help alleviate discomfort. Avoiding acidic foods and drinks and managing teeth grinding can also be beneficial.

3.4 Bad Breath (Halitosis): Causes and Tips for Fresh Breath

Bad breath, or halitosis, can be embarrassing and impact social interactions. It's often caused by bacteria in the mouth releasing sulfur compounds, leading to an unpleasant odor.

Causes: Poor oral hygiene, gum disease, dry mouth, certain foods, and smoking are common causes of bad breath. In some cases, underlying health conditions can also contribute.

Tips for Fresh Breath: Regular brushing and flossing, cleaning your tongue, staying hydrated, and avoiding tobacco can help combat bad breath. Chewing sugar-free gum and using mouthwash designed to target bad breath can provide temporary relief.

Understanding these common dental issues empowers you to take proactive steps in preventing them and seeking timely treatment if they arise. Regular dental check-ups play a vital role in catching and addressing these issues early, ensuring a healthier and more vibrant smile.

CHAPTER 4

Oral Hygiene Practices

Maintaining proper oral hygiene practices is essential for preserving the health of your teeth and gums.

4.1 Brushing Techniques: Choosing the Right Toothbrush and Toothpaste

Brushing your teeth is a cornerstone of oral hygiene, and using the right technique, along with suitable tools, can make a significant difference in maintaining tooth health.

Choosing the Right Toothbrush:
Select a toothbrush with soft bristles
to prevent enamel and gum irritation.
Choose a size that fits comfortably in
your mouth and allows easy access to
all areas of your teeth.

Choosing the Right Toothpaste: Opt
for toothpaste that contains fluoride, a
mineral that strengthens enamel and
helps prevent cavities. If you have
specific dental concerns like
sensitivity or gingivitis, look for
toothpaste formulated to address those
issues.

Brushing Technique:

1. Hold your toothbrush at a 45-
   degree angle to your gums.

2. Use gentle, circular motions to
   brush the outer surfaces of your
   teeth.

3. Brush the inner surfaces of your teeth using the same circular motions.

4. For the chewing surfaces, use a back-and-forth motion.

5. Brush your tongue to remove bacteria and maintain fresh breath.

Brushing Frequency: Brush your teeth at least twice a day, ideally in the morning and before bedtime. If possible, brush after meals to remove food particles and plaque.

4.2 Importance of Regular Flossing

Flossing is an often overlooked but crucial aspect of oral hygiene. It helps clean the areas between your teeth and along the gumline that your toothbrush might miss.

Why Flossing Matters: While brushing removes plaque from the surfaces of your teeth, flossing gets rid of food particles and plaque that accumulates between teeth and under the gumline. If not removed, these particles can contribute to cavities, gum disease, and bad breath.

Flossing Technique:

1. Use a piece of floss around 18 inches long.

2. Gently guide the floss between your teeth using a sawing motion. Avoid snapping the floss, as this can damage gums.

3. Curve the floss into a C-shape around each tooth and move it up and down to clean the sides.

4. Don't forget to floss behind your back teeth as well.

Flossing Frequency: Floss at least once a day, preferably before brushing your teeth at night. This ensures that your mouth is free from lingering food particles and plaque before you sleep.

Additional Tips:

- If traditional flossing is challenging, consider using floss picks or interdental brushes designed to clean between teeth.

- It's normal for gums to bleed a little when you first start flossing regularly. This usually indicates gum inflammation due to the presence of plaque. With consistent flossing, the bleeding should decrease over time.

Incorporating effective brushing and flossing techniques into your daily routine can significantly contribute to maintaining healthy teeth and gums. These simple practices, combined with regular dental check-ups, will help you enjoy a lifetime of good oral health.

4.3 Tongue Cleaning: Reducing Bacteria and Improving Oral Health

Cleaning your tongue is an often overlooked but crucial step in maintaining optimal oral health. The tongue's rough surface can harbor bacteria, food particles, and dead cells, contributing to bad breath and other oral issues.

Why Clean Your Tongue:

- **Reduce Bad Breath**: The majority of bad breath-causing bacteria reside on the back of the tongue. Cleaning your tongue can help minimize bad breath.

- **Improved Taste Sensation**: A clean tongue enhances your ability to taste food and enjoy flavors.

- **Reduced Bacterial Load**: Removing bacteria and debris from your tongue can help prevent oral infections and promote healthier gums.

Tongue Cleaning Technique:

1. Use a tongue scraper, tongue brush, or the back of your toothbrush.

2. Gently scrape or brush the surface of your tongue from the back to the front.

3. Rinse your mouth with water after tongue cleaning.

Frequency: Clean your tongue once a day, preferably in the morning or after brushing your teeth.

4.4 Mouthwash: Benefits and Proper Usage

Mouthwash, or oral rinse, is a liquid solution used to enhance oral hygiene. It can serve as a valuable addition to your oral care routine when used correctly.

Benefits of Mouthwash:

- **Fresh Breath**: Mouthwash can help temporarily mask bad breath and provide a refreshing feeling.

- **Reduced Plaque and Bacteria**: Certain mouthwashes contain antimicrobial agents that can help reduce bacteria and plaque in the mouth.

- **Gum Health**: Some mouthwashes are designed to target gum issues like gingivitis, promoting healthier gums.

- **Cavity Prevention**: Fluoride-containing mouthwashes can contribute to cavity prevention by strengthening enamel.

Proper Usage:

- **Follow Instructions**: Read and follow the manufacturer's instructions for the specific mouthwash you're using.

- **Timing**: Use mouthwash at a separate time from brushing to maximize its benefits. This can be in the morning or before bed.

- **Don't Swallow**: Spit out the mouthwash after rinsing. Avoid swallowing it, especially if it contains fluoride.

- **Children**: Supervise young children when using mouthwash to ensure they don't swallow it.

Choosing the Right Mouthwash:

- **Antiseptic Mouthwash**: Contains antimicrobial agents to kill bacteria. It's beneficial for reducing plaque and gingivitis.

- **Fluoride Mouthwash**: Contains fluoride to strengthen enamel and prevent cavities.

- **Cosmetic Mouthwash**: Primarily for freshening breath and providing a pleasant taste.

- **Prescription Mouthwash**: Some mouthwashes require a

prescription and are used for specific dental conditions.

Frequency: Mouthwash can be used once or twice a day, but it's not a substitute for brushing and flossing. Incorporate it as an additional step in your oral hygiene routine.

By incorporating tongue cleaning and mouthwash into your oral care practices, you can enhance the effectiveness of your routine and enjoy improved overall oral health. Remember that these practices should complement regular brushing and flossing, as well as regular visits to the dentist for comprehensive care.

CHAPTER 5

Healthy Dietary Habits for Strong Teeth

What you eat plays a significant role in maintaining strong and healthy teeth.

5.1 Foods That Promote Tooth Health: Calcium-Rich and Nutrient-Dense Choices

A balanced diet that includes foods rich in essential nutrients can contribute to strong teeth and gums.

Calcium-Rich Foods: Calcium is a vital mineral for building strong teeth and bones. Incorporate these calcium-rich foods into your diet:

- Dairy products: Milk, cheese, yogurt

- Leafy greens: Spinach, kale, collard greens

- Fortified foods: Calcium-fortified plant-based milk, cereals

Phosphorus-Rich Foods: Phosphorus works with calcium to maintain tooth health. Include these phosphorus sources:

- Lean proteins: Chicken, turkey, fish, eggs

- Nuts and seeds: Almonds, pumpkin seeds

Vitamin D Sources: Vitamin D aids in calcium absorption, crucial for tooth mineralization. Get vitamin D from:

- Fatty fish: Salmon, mackerel, sardines

- Fortified foods: Vitamin D-fortified milk, orange juice

Vitamin C-Rich Foods: Vitamin C supports gum health and collagen production. Opt for:

- Citrus fruits: Oranges, grapefruits, lemons

- Bell peppers

- Berries: Strawberries, blueberries

Water: Staying hydrated is essential for saliva production, which helps rinse away food particles and maintain oral health.

5.2 Foods to Limit: Sugars, Acids, and Starchy Snacks

Certain foods and beverages can contribute to dental issues if consumed in excess.

Sugary Foods and Drinks: Sugar feeds harmful bacteria in your mouth, leading to enamel erosion and cavities. Limit:

- Sugary snacks: Candies, cookies, cakes

- Sugary beverages: Soda, fruit juices, energy drinks

Acidic Foods: Acidic foods weaken enamel, making teeth susceptible to damage. Consume acidic foods in moderation:

- Citrus fruits

- Tomatoes

- Vinegar-based dressings

Starchy Snacks: Starchy foods can get trapped in the crevices of your teeth, promoting bacterial growth. Reduce intake of:

- Chips

- Crackers

- Bread

Sticky and Chewy Foods: These foods can cling to teeth, increasing the risk of cavities:

- Raisins

- Caramel candies

Tips for Dental-Friendly Eating:

- **Moderation**: Enjoy sugary and acidic foods in moderation and as part of meals, rather than snacking on them throughout the day.

- **Timing**: If consuming acidic foods, do so during mealtimes to minimize their impact on teeth.

- **Rinsing**: After eating sugary or acidic foods, rinse your mouth with water to help neutralize acids and remove particles.

- **Oral Hygiene**: Brush your teeth at least twice a day and floss daily to remove food particles and plaque.

Maintaining a balanced diet that supports your oral health not only benefits your teeth and gums but also contributes to your overall well-being. By making mindful food choices, you can promote strong teeth and reduce the risk of dental issues in the long run.

5.3 Drinking Water: Its Role in Oral Hygiene

Water is often referred to as the elixir of life, and its significance extends to oral hygiene as well. Staying adequately hydrated by drinking water throughout the day can have a positive impact on your oral health in various ways.

Rinsing Away Debris: Water helps to wash away food particles, bacteria, and debris from your mouth. This rinsing action helps prevent the accumulation of plaque and reduces the risk of cavities and gum disease.

Stimulating Saliva Production: Saliva is a natural defense mechanism for your teeth and gums. It contains enzymes that aid in digestion, minerals that remineralize teeth, and antibodies that fight harmful bacteria. Drinking water stimulates saliva production, promoting a healthier oral environment.

Neutralizing Acids: Water can help neutralize acids that are produced by bacteria in your mouth or that come from acidic foods and beverages. Acidic conditions can weaken enamel and lead to tooth erosion, so maintaining a balanced pH level is crucial.

Preventing Dry Mouth: Dehydration can lead to dry mouth, a condition where the mouth produces less saliva. Dry mouth can increase the risk of cavities and gum disease due to reduced protective saliva flow. Drinking water keeps your mouth moist and helps prevent dry mouth-related issues.

Fluoride Exposure: Many communities have fluoridated water supplies. Fluoride is a mineral that strengthens tooth enamel and makes teeth more resistant to decay. Drinking fluoridated water can provide a continuous supply of fluoride to your teeth, contributing to their health.

Tips for Optimal Water Consumption:

- Drink water throughout the day, and aim for at least 8 glasses (about 2 liters) or more, depending on your body's needs.

- Carry a reusable water bottle to encourage consistent hydration.

- Swish water around in your mouth after consuming acidic or sugary foods to help neutralize acids and minimize their impact on teeth.

- opt for tap water when possible, as it often contains fluoride that benefits your teeth.

while drinking water is beneficial for oral hygiene, it should complement other essential oral care practices such as regular brushing, flossing, and professional dental check-ups. By staying well-hydrated and maintaining

a comprehensive oral care routine,
you can contribute to the health and
longevity of your teeth and gums.

CHAPTER 6
Lifestyle Factors Affecting Tooth Health

Beyond your oral hygiene routine and diet, various lifestyle factors can significantly impact the health of your teeth and gums.

6.1 Smoking and Oral Health: Risks and Cessation

Smoking has detrimental effects on both your general health and your oral health. It can lead to severe dental issues and increase the risk of oral cancers.

Risks of Smoking for Oral Health:

- **Gum Disease**: Smoking weakens the immune system, making it harder for your body to fight gum infections. This can lead to gum disease, which can result in tooth loss if left untreated.

- **Tooth Discoloration**: Tobacco use can cause teeth to become discolored, staining them yellow or even brown.

- **Bad Breath**: Smoking contributes to bad breath and an unpleasant taste in the mouth.

- **Delayed Healing**: Smokers may experience slower healing after dental procedures, extractions, or surgeries.

- **Oral Cancer**: Smoking is a leading cause of oral cancer. It can affect the lips, mouth, throat, and even the tongue.

Cessation and Oral Health: Quitting smoking can greatly improve your oral health and reduce the risk of serious dental problems. Benefits include:

- **Gum Health**: Quitting smoking can slow the progression of gum disease and improve gum health.

- **Better Healing**: Your mouth's ability to heal after dental procedures will improve.

- **Fresh Breath**: Quitting smoking can lead to fresher

breath and a better taste in your mouth.

- **Reduced Cancer Risk**: Quitting smoking reduces the risk of oral cancer and other related health issues.

6.2 Impact of Stress on Teeth and Gums

Stress can affect your oral health in surprising ways. Chronic stress can contribute to several dental problems.

Teeth Grinding (Bruxism): Stress can lead to teeth grinding, often unconsciously during sleep. Bruxism can result in worn teeth, jaw pain, headaches, and even cracked teeth.

Gum Disease: Stress weakens the immune system, making it harder for your body to fend off infections, including gum disease.

Canker Sores and Cold Sores: Stress can trigger the appearance of canker sores or worsen cold sore outbreaks.

Neglecting Oral Hygiene: During times of stress, you may neglect your oral care routine, which can lead to the development of dental issues.

Coping Strategies:

- Practice stress management techniques, such as deep breathing, meditation, and exercise.

- Maintain a balanced lifestyle that includes sufficient sleep, a healthy diet, and regular physical activity.

- Be mindful of teeth grinding and consider wearing a nightguard if necessary.

Understanding how lifestyle factors can impact your oral health empowers you to make informed choices that support your overall well-being. Quitting smoking, managing stress, and maintaining a comprehensive oral care routine all contribute to healthier teeth and gums.

6.3 Effects of Alcohol Consumption on Oral Health

Alcohol consumption is another lifestyle factor that can have significant effects on oral health.

While moderate alcohol consumption may not have drastic effects on oral health, excessive or chronic alcohol use can lead to various dental issues.

Dry Mouth: Alcohol is dehydrating and can lead to reduced saliva production, causing dry mouth. Saliva plays a crucial role in rinsing away food particles, neutralizing acids, and maintaining a healthy oral environment.

Gum Disease: Excessive alcohol consumption weakens the immune system, making it harder for your body to fight infections, including gum disease. This can lead to inflamed gums, bleeding, and even tooth loss.

Tooth Erosion: Alcoholic beverages, especially those with high sugar or acid content, can contribute to enamel erosion. This can lead to tooth sensitivity, cavities, and other dental problems.

Oral Cancer: Heavy alcohol use, especially when combined with tobacco use, is a risk factor for oral cancer. Alcohol can irritate the tissues in your mouth, increasing the risk of cancerous growth.

Tips for Maintaining Oral Health with Alcohol Consumption:

1. **Moderation**: If you choose to consume alcohol, do so in moderation. Limiting your intake can help mitigate the negative effects on your oral health.

2. **Stay Hydrated**: Drink water along with alcoholic beverages to help counteract the dehydrating effects of alcohol.

3. **Oral Hygiene**: Maintain a consistent oral care routine that includes brushing, flossing, and rinsing with mouthwash. This can help minimize the impact of alcohol on your oral health.

4. **Limit Sugary and Acidic Drinks**: Choose alcoholic beverages with lower sugar and acid content to reduce the risk of tooth erosion.

5. **Regular Dental Check-ups**: Visit your dentist regularly for check-ups and cleanings. Your dentist can monitor your oral health and address any issues before they worsen.

6. **Avoid Tobacco**: If you're a smoker or use tobacco products, combining alcohol with tobacco significantly

increases the risk of oral health problems, including oral cancer.

Seek Professional Help if Needed: If you find it challenging to moderate your alcohol consumption or if you have concerns about its effects on your oral health, consider seeking guidance from a healthcare professional or counselor.

Understanding the effects of alcohol on oral health empowers you to make informed decisions that align with your overall well-being. By practicing moderation and maintaining a comprehensive oral care routine, you can support the health of your teeth and gums.

CHAPTER 7

Visiting the Dentist

Regular dental check-ups are a cornerstone of maintaining optimal oral health.

7.1 Importance of Regular Dental Check-ups

Routine dental check-ups play a crucial role in preventing dental issues, catching problems early, and maintaining a healthy smile.

Early Detection and Prevention: Regular dental visits allow your dentist to identify potential issues like cavities, gum disease, or oral cancer in their early stages. Early detection often leads to more effective and less invasive treatments.

Professional Cleaning: Even with diligent oral hygiene practices, plaque and tartar can accumulate over time. Professional dental cleanings remove these deposits, reducing the risk of cavities and gum disease.

Personalized Care: Your dentist can offer personalized advice tailored to your oral health needs. They can recommend proper brushing and flossing techniques, as well as suggest dietary and lifestyle changes to promote optimal oral health.

Monitoring Dental Health: Regular dental visits help track the progress of existing dental work, such as fillings, crowns, or implants. Your dentist can ensure these restorations are functioning well and address any issues early.

Gum Health: Your dentist will assess the health of your gums, measuring the depth of gum pockets and checking for signs of gum disease. Early intervention is key to preventing gum problems from worsening.

Oral Cancer Screening: Dentists are trained to recognize the early signs of oral cancer. Regular check-ups provide an opportunity for your dentist to perform an oral cancer screening, enhancing your chances of early detection and successful treatment.

7.2 What to Expect During a Dental Visit

Knowing what to expect during a dental visit can help ease any anxiety and ensure a productive appointment.

Health History Review: Your dentist will start by reviewing your medical and dental history. It's important to provide accurate information about any health conditions, medications, and past dental treatments.

Examination: Your dentist will conduct a thorough examination of your mouth, teeth, and gums. They will check for cavities, gum disease, bite alignment issues, and signs of oral cancer.

X-rays: Depending on your individual needs, your dentist may recommend dental X-rays to get a more comprehensive view of your oral health. X-rays can reveal hidden problems such as impacted teeth or bone loss.

Professional Cleaning: A dental hygienist will perform a professional cleaning, removing plaque and tartar buildup. They will also polish your teeth to remove surface stains and give your smile a fresh look.

Discussion and Recommendations: Your dentist will discuss their findings with you and recommend any necessary treatments or interventions. This is also an opportunity to ask questions and address any concerns you may have.

Treatment Planning: If additional treatments are needed, your dentist will create a treatment plan outlining the recommended procedures, their costs, and the expected timeline.

Scheduling Follow-up Visits: Based on your oral health status, your dentist will recommend the appropriate frequency of future dental check-ups. This could be every six months for routine care or more often for specific treatments.

Regular dental check-ups provide the foundation for a lifetime of good oral health. By maintaining these appointments, you are taking proactive steps to prevent dental issues and ensure that any problems are addressed early, leading to a healthier and more confident smile.

7.3 Professional Teeth Cleaning: Scaling and Polishing

Professional teeth cleaning, often referred to as dental prophylaxis, is a vital component of maintaining optimal oral health. This procedure involves two main steps: scaling and polishing. This section provides insights into what happens during a professional teeth cleaning session and its benefits.

Scaling:

Scaling is the process of removing plaque, tartar (calculus), and bacterial deposits from the surfaces of your teeth, both above and below the gumline. Even with regular brushing and flossing, certain areas can be challenging to clean effectively, leading to the accumulation of plaque and tartar. Dental professionals use specialized instruments to carefully remove these deposits, ensuring your teeth are clean and free from harmful bacteria.

Benefits of Scaling:

1. **Prevents Gum Disease**: Removing tartar and plaque buildup helps prevent gum disease by eliminating the source of inflammation and infection.

2. **Cavity Prevention**: Scaling removes bacteria that contribute to tooth decay, reducing the risk of cavities.

3. **Freshens Breath**: Bacteria-rich plaque can lead to bad breath. Scaling helps eliminate this source of odor.

4. **Healthier Gums**: Scaling
   promotes healthier gums by
   reducing inflammation and
   preventing pockets from forming
   between your teeth and gums.

Polishing:

After scaling, your teeth are polished
using a special paste and a rotating
brush or rubber cup. This process
helps remove surface stains and gives
your teeth a smoother, cleaner
appearance. Polishing also makes it
harder for plaque to adhere to the
tooth surfaces, aiding in oral hygiene
maintenance.

Benefits of Polishing:

1. **Enhanced Appearance**: Polishing
   removes stains caused by food,
   beverages, and habits like
   smoking, improving the
   appearance of your teeth.

2. **Smooth Tooth Surfaces**: Smooth tooth surfaces make it more difficult for plaque to accumulate, making your oral hygiene routine more effective.

3. **Cleaner Feeling**: After a professional polish, your teeth may feel cleaner and smoother.

Frequency:

For most people, professional teeth cleaning is recommended every six months. However, your dentist or dental hygienist may adjust the frequency based on your individual oral health needs. Some individuals with certain conditions, like gum disease, may require more frequent cleanings.

Post-Cleaning Care:

After a professional cleaning, continue practicing good oral hygiene at home by brushing your teeth at least twice a day and flossing daily. Maintaining these habits between professional cleanings will help keep your teeth and gums in excellent condition.

Professional teeth cleaning is a fundamental aspect of preventive dental care. By removing plaque, tartar, and stains, you not only promote a healthier smile but also reduce the risk of dental issues and enjoy the benefits of improved oral hygiene.

CHAPTER 8

Dental Products and Technologies

Advancements in dental products and technologies have provided us with various tools to maintain optimal oral health.

8.1 Electric vs. Manual Toothbrushes: Pros and Cons

The choice between an electric and a manual toothbrush ultimately comes down to personal preference and individual oral health needs. Both options have their own advantages and considerations.

Electric Toothbrushes: Pros

1. **Efficient Cleaning**: Electric toothbrushes often provide a more consistent and efficient cleaning compared to manual brushing, thanks to their rotating or oscillating bristle heads.

2. **Built-in Timers**: Many electric toothbrushes have built-in timers to ensure you brush for the recommended two minutes, promoting a thorough cleaning.

3. **Ease of Use**: Electric toothbrushes do a lot of the work for you, making them a good option for people with limited dexterity, such as children, the elderly, or individuals with certain physical conditions.

4. **Variety of Brushing Modes**:
    Some electric toothbrushes offer
    multiple brushing modes, such as
    sensitive, whitening, and gum care,
    catering to different oral health
    needs.

5. **Pressure Sensors**: Certain models
    come with pressure sensors that
    alert you if you're brushing too
    hard, helping prevent enamel
    erosion and gum irritation.

Electric Toothbrushes: Cons

1. **Cost**: Electric toothbrushes are
    generally more expensive upfront
    than manual toothbrushes, and
    replacement brush heads can also
    add to the long-term cost.

2. **Battery Charging**: Electric
    toothbrushes require charging, so
    you need to ensure they are
    adequately powered before use.

3. **Portability**: Electric toothbrushes might be less portable compared to manual brushes, especially when traveling or if you don't have access to a charging station.

Manual Toothbrushes: Pros

1. **Affordability**: Manual toothbrushes are more budget-friendly upfront and don't require ongoing expenses for replacement brush heads or batteries.

2. **Portability**: Manual toothbrushes are easy to carry and use anywhere without needing to worry about battery life or charging.

3. **Simplicity**: There's no learning curve with a manual toothbrush; anyone can use it without needing to understand different settings.

Manual Toothbrushes: Cons

1. **Brushing Technique**: Achieving a
    consistent and efficient brushing
    technique can be more challenging
    with a manual toothbrush
    compared to an electric one.

2. **Limited Features**: Manual
    toothbrushes lack the built-in
    timers, pressure sensors, and
    multiple brushing modes found in
    many electric models.

Choosing the Right Brush for You:

Consider your individual needs and
preferences when choosing between
an electric and a manual toothbrush. If
you have specific oral health
concerns, such as gum disease or
sensitivity, consult your dentist for
personalized recommendations.

Ultimately, the most important factor
is maintaining a consistent and
thorough oral hygiene routine,

regardless of the type of toothbrush you use. Regular brushing, flossing, and professional dental check-ups are key to achieving and maintaining optimal oral health.

8.2 Choosing the Right Mouthwash and Dental Floss

Choosing the Right Mouthwash:

Mouthwash, or oral rinse, can be a valuable addition to your oral hygiene routine. There are different types of mouthwashes available, each serving specific purposes. Here are some considerations for choosing the right mouthwash:

1. **Fluoride Content**: If cavity prevention is a priority, opt for a fluoride-containing mouthwash. Fluoride helps strengthen tooth enamel and prevent cavities.

2. **Antiseptic or Antibacterial**: Antiseptic mouthwashes contain ingredients that can help kill bacteria and reduce plaque. They are beneficial for maintaining gum health and freshening breath.

3. **Alcohol-Free Options**: Some people prefer alcohol-free mouthwashes to avoid dry mouth or irritation. Alcohol-free options can still provide effective oral care.

4. **Specific Concerns**: Some mouthwashes are formulated to address specific concerns, such as sensitivity, gum disease, or dry

mouth. Choose a mouthwash that aligns with your needs.

5. **Cosmetic Mouthwash**: Cosmetic mouthwashes primarily freshen breath and provide a pleasant taste. They may not offer the same therapeutic benefits as other types.

6. **Prescription Mouthwash**: In some cases, your dentist may prescribe a specialized mouthwash for specific oral health conditions. Follow your dentist's recommendations.

Choosing the Right Dental Floss:

Dental floss is essential for cleaning between teeth and along the gumline, where toothbrushes can't reach effectively. Here's how to choose the right dental floss:

1. **Type of Floss**: There are different types of dental floss, including traditional floss, dental tape, floss picks, and interdental brushes. Choose the type that feels most comfortable and effective for you.

2. **Thickness**: Dental floss comes in various thicknesses. Thicker floss may be more suitable if you have wider gaps between your teeth, while thinner floss is better for tight spaces.

3. **Wax Coating**: Some floss is coated with wax to make it glide more easily between teeth. This can be particularly helpful if you have tight contacts.

4. **Flavor**: Some dental floss options come in different flavors to make the flossing experience more pleasant.

5. **Floss Picks**: Floss picks are pre-threaded with a short strand of floss, making them convenient for on-the-go use. They're also useful for people with dexterity challenges.

6. **Interdental Brushes**: Interdental brushes are small brushes designed to clean between teeth. They are suitable for individuals with larger gaps between teeth.

Personalized Recommendations:

Your dentist or dental hygienist can offer personalized recommendations for mouthwash and dental floss based on your oral health needs and preferences. If you have specific concerns, such as sensitive gums or orthodontic appliances, consult your dental professional for guidance.

Regular use of mouthwash and dental floss, in addition to brushing and professional dental cleanings, contributes to a comprehensive oral hygiene routine that supports your overall oral health.

Advancements in dental technology have introduced a range of tools and devices that can enhance your oral hygiene routine.

8.3 Role of Technology: Toothbrush Apps, Water Flossers, and More

Toothbrush Apps:

Toothbrush apps are smartphone applications designed to improve your brushing technique and promote better oral hygiene habits. These apps often connect to smart toothbrushes equipped with sensors that track your brushing movements. Some features of toothbrush apps include:

1. **Brushing Timers**: Apps ensure you brush for the recommended two minutes by providing a timer that guides your brushing session.

2. **Pressure Sensors**: If your toothbrush has pressure sensors, the app can alert you if you're brushing too hard, helping prevent enamel erosion and gum damage.

3. **Brushing Feedback**: Toothbrush apps can provide real-time feedback on your brushing technique, helping you address areas you might be missing.

4. **Customized Routines**: Some apps allow you to create personalized

brushing routines based on your specific oral health needs.

Water Flossers:

Water flossers, also known as oral irrigators, use a stream of water to remove food particles and bacteria from between teeth and along the gumline. These devices can be particularly helpful for people with braces, bridges, or other dental work that makes traditional flossing challenging.

1. **Gentle and Effective**: Water flossers are gentle on the gums and can effectively clean areas that traditional floss might miss.

2. **Variability in Pressure**: Many water flossers allow you to adjust the water pressure to your comfort level, making it suitable for different oral sensitivities.

3. **Plaque Removal**: Water flossers
    can help remove plaque and debris
    from areas that are hard to reach
    with traditional floss.

Electric Toothbrushes with Bluetooth Connectivity:

Some electric toothbrushes come with
Bluetooth connectivity, allowing them
to sync with smartphone apps. This
technology adds an interactive
element to your oral care routine:

1. **Brushing Data**: The toothbrush
    can send data to the app about your
    brushing habits, duration, and
    areas you've brushed.

2. **Guided Brushing**: The app can
    provide guided brushing sessions,
    ensuring you cover all areas of
    your mouth evenly.

3. **Progress Tracking**: You can track your brushing progress over time and receive recommendations for improvement.

UV Sanitizers:

UV sanitizers are devices designed to sanitize toothbrush heads using ultraviolet light. They can help eliminate bacteria and germs that may be present on your toothbrush after use.

Smart Toothbrushes:

Some toothbrushes come equipped with sensors and technology that provide real-time feedback on your brushing technique. They can guide you to brush at the correct angle and ensure even coverage.

While these technological advancements can enhance your oral hygiene routine, it's important to remember that technology should complement rather than replace fundamental practices like regular brushing, flossing, and professional dental check-ups. If you're interested in incorporating dental technology into your routine, consult your dentist or dental hygienist for recommendations based on your individual oral health needs.

CHAPTER 9

Emergency Tooth Care

Knowing how to handle dental emergencies is crucial for minimizing damage and ensuring prompt treatment.

9.1 Dealing with a Knocked-Out Tooth

A knocked-out tooth, also known as an avulsed tooth, requires immediate attention to increase the chances of successful reimplantation. Here's what to do:

1. **Handle the Tooth Carefully**: Hold the tooth by the crown (the visible part) and avoid touching the roots. Rinse it gently with water if it's dirty, but don't scrub or remove any attached tissue fragments.

2. **Keep the Tooth Moist**: If possible, place the tooth back in its socket. If this isn't possible, keep the tooth moist by placing it in milk, a saline solution, or even saliva. Avoid using tap water, as it may damage the cells on the tooth root.

3. **Seek Immediate Dental Care**: Time is critical. Get to a dentist or an emergency room as soon as possible, ideally within 30 minutes. The dentist may be able to reimplant the tooth successfully.

4. **Avoid Touching the Root**: The root of the tooth is fragile and sensitive. Avoid touching it to preserve the cells necessary for reattachment.

9.2 Managing Toothache and Pain

Toothaches can range from mild discomfort to severe pain. If you're experiencing toothache or dental pain, consider these steps:

1. **Rinse with Warm Water**: Gently rinse your mouth with warm water to clean the area around the painful tooth.

2. **Floss Gently**: Sometimes toothache is caused by food particles stuck between teeth. Carefully floss to remove any

debris, but be gentle to avoid injuring the gums.

3. **Pain Relief**: Over-the-counter pain relievers like ibuprofen can help alleviate toothache. Follow the recommended dosage and instructions.

4. **Avoid Hot or Cold Foods**: Extreme temperatures can worsen tooth sensitivity. Stick to lukewarm or room temperature foods and drinks.

5. **Avoid Applying Aspirin**: Do not place aspirin directly on the painful tooth or gums. It can cause tissue damage and won't provide effective relief.

6. **See a Dentist**: If the pain persists, worsens, or is accompanied by swelling, pus, or fever, see a dentist as soon as possible. These

could be signs of an infection or other serious dental issue.

Immediate Dental Care:

If you're experiencing severe pain, bleeding, or a dental emergency, contact your dentist or an emergency dental clinic for advice. Dental professionals can provide guidance over the phone and arrange for urgent care if needed. It's important to address dental emergencies promptly to prevent further complications and ensure the best possible outcome.

9.3 Temporary Solutions Until You See a Dentist

When faced with dental emergencies, temporary solutions can help manage discomfort and prevent further damage until you can see a dentist.

Lost Filling or Crown:

If a filling or crown falls out, you can take these steps:

1. **Save the Restoration**: If possible, keep the lost filling or crown. Your dentist might be able to reattach it.

2. **Temporary Sealant**: Pharmacies sell temporary dental cement. Gently clean the tooth and restoration, and apply the cement to hold the restoration in place temporarily.

3. **Avoid Chewing**: Be cautious when chewing on the affected side to prevent further damage.

Chipped or Broken Tooth:

For a chipped or broken tooth, consider the following:

1. **Rinse**: Gently rinse your mouth
    with warm water to clean the area.

2. **Cold Compress**: Apply a cold
    compress to reduce swelling.

3. **Avoid Chewing**: Avoid chewing
    on the affected side to prevent
    worsening the damage.

4. **Dental Wax**: If the chipped area is
    sharp and irritating, you can place
    dental wax over it to protect your
    tongue and cheeks.

Loose or Dislodged Tooth:

If a tooth becomes loose or partially
dislodged, try these steps:

1. **Gently Reposition**: Gently try to
    reposition the tooth back into its
    original place. Bite down to keep it
    in position.

2. **Soft Diet**: Stick to a soft diet and avoid putting pressure on the affected tooth.

3. **Cold Compress**: Apply a cold compress to manage swelling.

Abscess or Swelling:

If you notice an abscess or swelling, take the following precautions:

1. **Warm Saltwater Rinse**: Rinse your mouth with warm saltwater to help alleviate pain and draw out pus.

2. **Over-the-Counter Pain Relievers**: If safe for you, take over-the-counter pain relievers as directed.

3. **Avoid Heat**: Avoid using heat on the affected area as it can worsen inflammation.

These are temporary solutions to manage discomfort and prevent further damage. It's crucial to see a dentist as soon as possible for proper diagnosis and treatment. Dental issues can worsen if left untreated, so even if the pain subsides, it's important to have a professional evaluation. If you're unsure about how to handle a dental emergency, contact your dentist or an emergency dental clinic for guidance.

CHAPTER 10

Building Lifelong Tooth Health Habits

Maintaining optimal tooth health requires establishing lifelong oral care habits. We will focus on creating a personalized oral care routine and the importance of motivation and consistency for successful tooth health.

10.1 Creating a Personalized Oral Care Routine

Creating a personalized oral care routine is essential for meeting your individual dental needs. Here's how to develop an effective routine:

1. **Consult Your Dentist**: Start by consulting your dentist. They can assess your oral health, identify any specific concerns, and provide personalized recommendations.

2. **Brushing**: Brush your teeth at least twice a day for two minutes each time. Use a fluoride toothpaste and a soft-bristle toothbrush. Consider using an electric toothbrush for efficient cleaning.

3. **Flossing**: Floss your teeth daily to clean between teeth and along the gumline. Choose dental floss that suits your preferences and needs.

4. **Mouthwash**: If recommended by your dentist, incorporate mouthwash into your routine.

Choose one that addresses your specific oral health concerns.

5. **Dietary Choices**: Consume a balanced diet rich in nutrient-dense foods that support tooth health. Limit sugary and acidic foods and beverages.

6. **Hydration**: Drink plenty of water throughout the day to help rinse away food particles and maintain a moist oral environment.

7. **Regular Dental Visits**: Schedule regular dental check-ups and cleanings as recommended by your dentist. These visits are crucial for early detection and preventive care.

8. **Oral Hygiene Products**: Choose dental products that suit your needs, such as toothbrushes, toothpaste, and floss. Consult your

dentist if you're unsure about the best options.

9. **Oral Health Monitoring**: Pay attention to any changes in your oral health, such as bleeding gums, tooth sensitivity, or bad breath. Address these issues promptly.

10.2 Motivation and Consistency: Keys to Successful Tooth Health

Maintaining good oral health requires both motivation and consistency. Here's how to stay motivated and build habits:

1. **Set Goals**: Set specific goals for your oral health, such as reducing plaque buildup, improving gum health, or achieving whiter teeth.

2. **Visualize Success**: Imagine the benefits of optimal oral health, including a confident smile and reduced risk of dental issues.

3. **Use Reminders**: Set reminders on your phone or place visual cues (sticky notes, dental products) to prompt you to brush, floss, and use mouthwash.

4. **Make It Enjoyable**: Find ways to make your oral care routine enjoyable. Play your favorite music, listen to an audiobook, or incorporate mindfulness.

5. **Track Progress**: Keep track of your progress, such as tracking how often you brush and floss. Seeing improvements can be motivating.

6. **Celebrate Achievements**: Celebrate milestones in your oral

care journey. Treat yourself to a small reward for sticking to your routine.

7. **Accountability**: Share your oral health goals with a friend or family member who can provide encouragement and hold you accountable.

8. **Be Patient**: Habits take time to form. Be patient with yourself and focus on gradual improvement.

Building lifelong tooth health habits requires dedication and effort, but the rewards are well worth it. Consistently following a personalized oral care routine and staying motivated will contribute to a healthier smile, improved overall well-being, and reduced dental problems over time.